LABOUR WARD RULES

LABOUR WARD RULES

TOBY FAY

Consultant Obstetrician and Gynaecologist,
Nottingham City Hospital NHS Trust,
UK

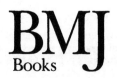

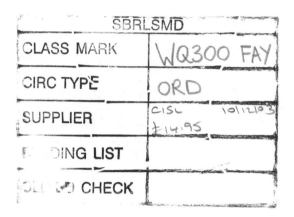
© BMJ Books 2001
BMJ Books is an imprint of the BMJ Publishing Group

First published in 2001
Second impression 2003
by BMJ Books, BMA House, Tavistock Square,
London WC1H 9JR

www.bmjbooks.com

British Library Cataloguing in Publication Data

A catalogue record for this book is available
from the British Library

ISBN 0–7279–1635–1

Typeset by Newgen Imaging Systems (P) Ltd, Chennai, India
Printed and bound in Spain by Graphycems, Navarra

Contents

Induction of labour

2 Fetal monitoring

3 Operative deliveries

Instrumental

Caesarean section

Vaginal trauma

4 Complex deliveries

Breech

Twin deliveries

Shoulder dystocia

5 Obstetric haemorrhage and shock

6 Infection

7 Preterm deliveries

Preface

This book is not a textbook for trainee midwives or obstetricians and it assumes a certain amount of knowledge and understanding of the physiology, sociology, and pathology associated with childbirth in the twenty-first century in Britain. Experience counts for a lot in obstetrics when there are complications or unusual presentations of common problems. But what is experience if not a collection of anecdotal personal experiences of clinical problems or situations?

This book brings together a set of basic rules to guide trainees in the labour ward when the going gets tough. No apology is made for the fact that at times the rules may seem prescriptive but one of the aims of the rules is to try to keep women, babies, and clinicians out of trouble. The rules are evidence based where evidence is available, but otherwise it is a mixture of common sense and experience. There is also space throughout the book for readers to write down their own labour ward rules.

Learning from one's experiences is an essential part of clinical maturity. The old adage goes: "Let every man be your teacher", and it means that decision-makers teach observers how to do things or, should the outcome be sub-optimal, perhaps how not to do things. Hopefully, this book will teach how "to do things" but in the event that clinicians decide not to follow these basic rules and can justify a different approach, then the book would have achieved another of its aims. That is, to have made trainees think carefully about their actions and interventions and to monitor or audit the consequences of those actions.

Introduction

By way of introduction and before starting with the labour ward rules, here are some thoughts on maternity care for consideration.

What we do – the maternity process

If one were to analyse the processes that occur during the clinical management of any labour by midwives and obstetricians, the activities could be simplified and categorised into three basic components:

- assessments
- record keeping
- interventions

This process has been previously referred to as *the obstetric process* (see Figure 1) but can rightly be expanded to include midwifery practice as well.

Assessments

Assessments are performed by obtaining a history, performing an examination, and reviewing the results from investigations or tests. Assessments can be either subjective or objective and obstetricians need to be familiar with test performance in relation to pregnancy. Observational statistics qualify test performance using the parameters: sensitivity, specificity, and predictive values (positive and negative). In addition, most of these assessments are prone to inter- and intra-observer variation. Midwives and obstetricians perform large numbers of assessments at any one visit or consultation, e.g. maternal height, weight, blood pressure, urinalysis, fundal height, fetal heart rate movements, responses to stimuli, ultrasound biometry, biophysical profiles etc.

Record keeping

The observations obtained from assessments must be recorded clearly, concisely, and accurately for good communications and to demonstrate "best practice" (see below), and when review of a case is necessary either for audit, complaints procedures or litigation. During labour records of assessments are recorded on the partograph. This

Introduction

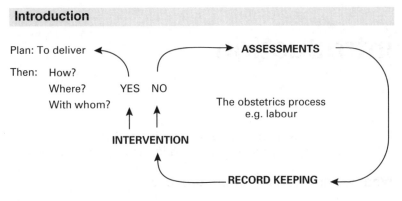

Figure 1   The obstetric process.

process has been shown to aid in the differentiation of normal from abnormal labour and identification of the women likely to require intervention. The timed entries should be written in black ink to enable accurate reproduction and every free-text entry should be dated and timed. Antenatal notes, either hand-held or hospital-based, must be available for scrutiny in order to review the antenatal assessments that may influence the management of the labour. The planning and performance of interventions similarly needs to be recorded. These records may serve to demonstrate that there has been no neglect of duty by maternity care providers.

Interventions

An intervention is an action that is required to reduce negative outcomes in pregnancy or childbirth and is usually in the form of a therapy, either medical or surgical. Normal labour is a physiological process and obstetricians do not need to intervene unduly. Interventions should be evidence based wherever possible and with an awareness of their level of effectiveness (Table 1).

When no evidence is available and there are randomised trials ongoing to resolve the issue, then consideration should be given to entering the woman in appropriate trials, for example: GRIT (Growth Restriction Intervention Trial). Two common obstetric interventions performed in labour are its induction or augmentation and operative deliveries.

The outcome from any intervention is time-dependent (Table 2). An intervention that results in a timely delivery for a fetal bradycardia by Caesarean section with a healthy outcome could be contrasted with the same intervention performed too late and results in a fresh stillbirth. An obstetrician should be continually questioning the

Table 1 Effectiveness of interventions.

Classification of effectiveness	Examples of interventions
1. Beneficial	Antibiotic during labour for women colonised with group B Streptococcus
2. Likely to be beneficial	External cephalic version for breech presentation in early labour with intact membranes
3. Balance between beneficial and adverse	Induction of labour for pre-labour rupture of membranes at term
4. Unknown effectiveness	Magnesium sulphate and calcium channel blockers to stop preterm labour
5. Unlikely to be beneficial	Caesarean section for non-active herpes simplex before or at the onset of labour
6. Ineffectual or harmful	Elective delivery for pre-labour rupture of membranes preterm

Adapted from Chalmers I, Enkin M, Keirse MJNC. *Effective care in pregnancy and childbirth*, Oxford University Press, 1991.

timing and necessity of an obstetric intervention: "Do I have to intervene or can I wait?". If the answer to that question should be that intervention is inappropriate, then further assessments must be performed to confirm fetal and maternal well-being. If the answer should be that the intervention is appropriate (e.g. delivery of the baby), then the next questions to be answered would be: How? With what? Where? When? and With whom? That is, to perform the intervention it must be planned and thought through.

Interventions have become more complex with the dictate from "Changing Childbirth", which has encouraged women to take control of their destiny and to give them choice. In other words, women can choose to have an intervention and, for example, elect to have a

Table 2 Qualities of obstetric interventions.

1. **Bimodal: Yes or No**
   If NO, go back and make more assessments (see Figure 1)
2. **Time-dependent**
   To be effective must be timed appropriately
3. **Should be evidence based where available**
   If no evidence, then reason and common sense should prevail
4. **Outcomes and interventions must be audited**
   To detect and reduce unnecessary interventions and to monitor their complications
5. **No interventions for pregnancy-related physiological changes**
6. **Based on necessity**
   To procure a good outcome

Caesarean birth. This brings us to the concept that interventions in maternity care can be seen as:

- **Needed**: interventions that are necessary to procure satisfactory pregnancy outcome, generally determined by medical staff.
- **Wanted**: interventions that are perceived by women to be necessary for a satisfactory pregnancy outcome.
- **Supplied**: whether interventions are provided by the health care resources provided by the state in which the woman resides.

These three entities are represented in a Venn diagram which defines seven areas (see Figure 2).

The skill required of the carers is they have to counsel and help the woman and her partner with their choice and hopefully direct them to make the right choice for them with all issues considered (Area 7). If, in the opinion of the carers, women were to make the wrong choice

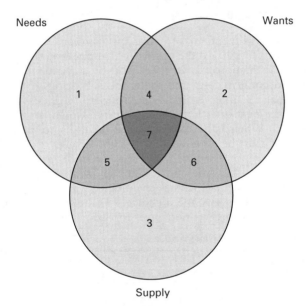

Figure 2
1. Intervention is needed but is neither wanted nor supplied.
2. Intervention is wanted but is neither needed nor supplied.
3. Intervention is supplied but is neither needed nor wanted.
4. Intervention is needed and wanted but not supplied.
5. Intervention is needed and supplied but not wanted.
6. Intervention is wanted and supplied but not needed.
7. Intervention is needed, wanted, and supplied.

(Area 6), then the women need to be informed of all the possible consequences of their chosen intervention and it should be explained that they might not necessarily need that intervention for satisfactory pregnancy outcome. The choice to refuse an intervention that has been deemed to be needed by maternity staff must be respected, but careful documentation is essential (Area 5). At the end of the counselling an amicable, sensible, and informed agreement should be reached.

How to survive

Life is tough on labour wards now, with patient expectations soaring to unreachable heights, increasing complaints and litigation, re-evaluation, suspensions, Ombudsman's enquiries, satisfaction surveys, and so it goes on. However, maternity care remains an immensely satisfying occupation and many, many women are very grateful and satisfied with the care they receive, and the perinatal mortality has never been so low. The challenge for those in maternity care is to practise to the highest possible standard of care and to be able to demonstrate the same by the keeping of concise and accurate medical records of events around the birth. To practise defensive medicine is negative and may result in unnecessary interventions and is a disservice to the mothers and babies. Be positive: "Best practice; not defensive medicine".

In addition to this, proper attitudes and communication skills are essential for the success and satisfaction of modern midwives and obstetricians.

Another issue which impacts on maternity care is the apportionment of skill and needs, and so: "It is not the healthy who need a doctor but the sick" (Matthew 9: v12).

One of the objectives of antenatal care is to determine the problems that may be relevant and to apportion appropriate care. Women who do not have any pregnancy problems do not need to be attended by a medical practitioner. This is the discrepancy between the developed and the developing world. In the developed world, private medicine leads to possible inappropriate mix of women's needs and supply of medical expertise which may lead to unnecessary intervention and unwise or ill-considered choice (Area 6). While in poor countries with no funded health care the necessary interventions may not supplied to meet the needs of the women (Areas 1 and 4; possibly 2) and choice may not be available and interventions could be enforced inappropriately (Area 3).

The rule of Ps

Question: What vegetable do you think of every time you enter the labour ward?

Answer: Peas

It is amazing how many words in midwives' and obstetricians' vocabulary begin with the letter "P". But it seems that this phenomenon has been observed in other branches of medical practice.[1] The very process itself heads a long list.

Consider the importance of each one:

Parturition
Powers
Passenger
Passages
Presenting part
Presentation
Position
Progress
Partogram
Prostaglandins
Prolonged labour
Persistent occipito-posterior
Posture
Pressures (blood, intrauterine, emotional, staff)
Partners
Practitioners
Pushing
Pulling
Pelvis
Pain
Perineum
Pudendal nerve block
Placenta praevia
Postpartum haemorrhage
pH
Perinatal morbidity and mortality

[1]Hayden GF. Alliteration in medicine: a puzzling profusion of Ps. *BMJ* 1999; **319**: 1605–8.

Paediatrician
Passing urine
Pyelonephritis
Prevention of adverse outcomes and complications
Preterm labour
Pre-eclampsia
Protect airways
Pulmonary embolism
Puerperium
Prolactin
Puerperal sepsis
Penicillin
Postnatal depression
Prolapse
Prosecution

Communications

The cornerstone of good maternity care is good communications. However, it often ends up being the stumbling block that falls into complaint and litigation procedures. Good communications consists of face-to-face, frank discussions with the women and their partners about their needs and wants, assessment results and their meaning and interpretation, and interventions and their aims and implications. Communication also extends laterally with our colleagues, whether they be anaesthetists, paediatricians, laboratory staff, or whoever; and vertically with the seniors to pass on clear and concise assessments of problems or planned interventions, and to experienced seniors to instruct and teach those less experienced members of the team. An Italian saying goes: "*Male non fare, paura non avere*", which can be translated in the context of this book as "Do no harm, and have no fear". There is no doubt that many obstetric interventions require skills that are achieved through experience and hard work and that these skills must be passed on to trainees. "Do no harm" needs to be properly balanced with the notion, "have the courage of your conviction". This will result in best practice and satisfying and good outcomes.

But let us choose the vocabulary well and not be misinterpreted; we must change from denotation and medical terminology to connotation without loss of accuracy. "Abortion" has changed to miscarriage; "intrauterine growth retardation" to intrauterine growth restriction. Let us speak of birth rather than delivery and shed forever the words "failed" and "failure". How can we sell ourselves in maternity care if we use these dreadful terms: "failed induction of labour", "failure to progress" and worst of all: "failed forceps/ventouse". Moreover, the women may think that they have failed, which is not true.

1 Labour

The important parts are the Passages, Powers, Passenger, and Placenta

The three Ps (Passages, Powers, Passenger) represents nothing new in the teaching of obstetrics to medical and midwifery staff. In this rule, a fourth P has been added to reinforce the fact that the delivery or birth process is not complete until the placenta has been safely delivered in its entirety AND the uterus is contracted and remains so. The successful birth of a healthy baby is a miraculous and joyous event but the care of the mother remains unfinished until all the products of the conception have been safely delivered. The mother can rest while the uterus continues to contract unabated to protect her from postpartum haemorrhage.

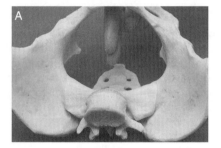

SPNP: sacral promontory, not palpable.

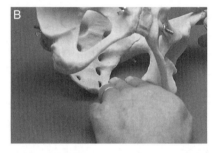

SSL2F: sacrospinous ligaments, two fingers.

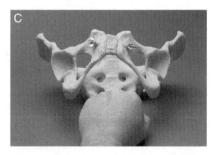

ITD4K: inter-tuberous distance, four knuckles.

SPNP/SSL2F/ITD4K

Most forms of pelvimetry are of limited value in predicting the outcome of the very dynamic process which is called labour. This is because pelvimetry relates to "the passages", one of the variables involved in the process of parturition; and of the three (or four) Ps, the shape and dimensions of the pelvis display the least variation. Nevertheless, a knowledge of the properties of the pelvis is important to the understanding of labour.

This cryptic-looking rule is something an old obstetrician used to write in his patient's notes, and when deciphered it provides quite a good summary of clinical pelvimetry. The problem with clinical pelvimetry is that it depends on the size of the assessor's fingers and hands. This clinical assessment provides some subjective information about the smallest pelvic diameters and assumes that all the other diameters are larger.

SPNP: Sacral promontory, not palpable This is the gynaecological conjugate or a measure of the anterio-posterior diameter of the pelvic inlet, the smallest diameter of the inlet; the largest is the transverse diameter.

SSL2F: Sacrospinous ligaments, two fingers The ischial spines are the narrowest part of the pelvis, and if the sacrospinous ligaments accommodate less than two fingers it means the sacrum and ischial spines are in close proximity thus allowing less from for rotation of the presenting part.

ITD4K: Inter-tuberous distance, four knuckles The distance between the ischial tuberosities represents the transverse diameter of the pelvic outlet and the smallest diameter (the width of one's fist, i.e. four knuckles or 10 cm), the largest diameter of which is the anterio-posterior diameter. The smaller the inter-tuberous distance, the narrower the sub-pubic arch of the pelvic outlet.

The largest diameter of the pelvis rotates through 90° from inlet to outlet, and as it rotates it also changes direction 90° from down to forward in the sagittal plane to permit the presenting part of the fetus under the pubic symphysis.

Exception

The are racial differences in pelvic shapes and dimensions, the best example of which is the African pelvis which has a high angle of inclination and is shallow.

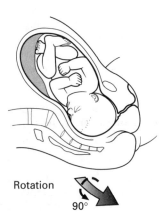

Descent and flexion

Rotation
90°

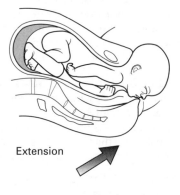

Extension

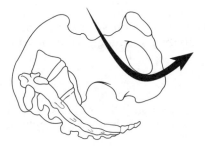

Labour: The powers

Uterine contractions represent the work (labour) required to overcome three levels of pelvic resistance to achieve a spontaneous birth:

- the cervix
- the pelvic floor (levators ani)
- the perineum

These correlate with the three main actions or mechanisms applied to the fetal head and used to describe the birth process:

- descent
- rotation
- extension

These processes occur in sequence but not necessarily one after the other, and may even occur simultaneously.

Progress, progress; all is progress

The first stage of labour can be likened to a vehicle going up a hill: the steepness of the hill is the amount of pelvic resistance, the engine is the uterine contractions, and the vehicle is the fetus. The progress is the rate at which the vehicle goes up the hill and in labour is assessed by cervical dilatation, descent, and rotation of the presenting part, i.e. the head. All the parameters of progress are recorded on the partogram with appropriate "alert" and "action" lines.[1]

If progress is unsatisfactory then an intervention will be necessary to limit the length of time in labour to enhance uterine work, usually in the case of nulliparous woman, oxytocin augmentation or to use the motoring analogy: "putting the foot down on the accelerator".

---

[1]World Health Organisation Maternal and Safe Motherhood Programme. WHO partograph in management of labour. *Lancet* 1994; **343**: 1399–404.

Partners are important, especially supportive and helpful ones

The active management of labour described above has to be supported by an important psychological element of encouragement of either a qualified or unqualified companion throughout labour.

In a meta-analysis of 10 randomised trials containing over 3000 women it appears that it is this support which affords benefits to labouring women in that it seemed to reduce the need for analgesia and operative delivery and to improve fetal outcome.[1]

[1]Thornton JG and Lilford RJ. Active management of labour: current knowledge and research issues. *BMJ* 1994; **309**: 366–9.

Partogram × 2 pages = perinatal mortality;
Partogram × 3 pages = maternal mortality

This means that prolonged labours are dangerous to both the mother and the baby, and in modern practice are not tolerated. Early intervention and augmentation are essential to ensure that the labour progresses. Maternal and fetal exhaustion and distress, hypoxia, and infection are undesirable consequences that are best avoided.

Uterine inertia in the 1st stage = uterine inertia in the 2nd stage = uterine inertia in the 3rd stage of labour

Uncoordinated, infrequent, and inefficient uterine contractions mean a prolonged first stage of labour (primary dysfunctional labour), with slow or no progress. Appropriately timed intervention with oxytocics (with appropriate doses), will prevent the all too common and dreadful scenario: "Caesarean section for failure to progress". Who has failed? The birth attendants have failed to identify and intervene to correct an abnormal labour and lack of progress.

When progress is re-established, however, be on guard for two problems in the other stages of labour. The first is delay in the second stage, necessitating instrumental delivery; and the second is a predisposition in the third stage to primary postpartum haemorrhage as a consequence of uterine atony.

So get the uterus contracting and keep it going well after the baby has been delivered.

Late secondary arrest will test the best

Secondary arrest is a serious abnormal first stage labour pattern that results in lack of progress and which may suggest relative or absolute cephalo-pelvic disproportion. The greater the cervical dilatation at which the arrest of progress occurs, the more serious the potential problem for the fetus. The metabolic reserves, stored up in the antenatal period to help the fetus to cope with the relative hypoxia associated with uterine contractions, may become depleted and risk metabolic decompensation, anoxia, and acidosis.

For the obstetrician it means a complete review of the labour and a carefully timed management plan which may involve reassessment of the labour in 30–60 minutes. Relative cephalo-pelvic disproportion due to an occipito-posterior position, with adequate fetal reserves, may be overcome by judicious use of oxytocin. Absolute disproportion is an indication for immediate delivery and oxytocin is contraindicated.

Size 8 pelvis, size 6 baby: No problem;
Size 6 pelvis, size 8 baby: No go;
Size 7 pelvis, size 7 baby: Don't know

The third variable that influences the outcome of any labour is the fetus (the passenger). The three fetal parameters that are important are the size, position, and attitude of the presenting part (in this case the head).

The rule given above is the obstetric rule of relativity. It explains the relationship between the maternal pelvis and the baby (or fetal head) and assumes efficient uterine contractions. Most labours represent the normal physiological process of parturition (P8/B6). While many fewer are pathological and obstructed (P6/B8). The remainder represent a tighter fit (P7/B7), and the mode of delivery will depend on the uterine response to more work and the position and attitude of the fetal head as it descends into the pelvis and meets the musculature of the pelvic floor.

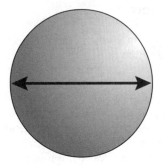

Hen's egg:
viewed from above

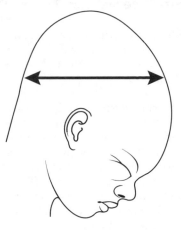

Occipito-anterior position
Attitude: flexed

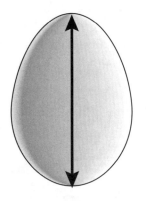

Hen's egg:
viewed from the side

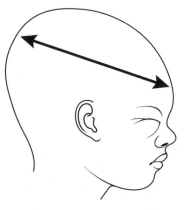

Occipito-posterior position
Attitude: deflexed

A baby's head is like a hen's egg.

The fetal head is shaped like an egg

There is not so much a rule as an observation from nature that explains the concept of fetal attitude and the different cephalic diameters.

The fetal head has a large longitudinal diameter and a small vertical diameter and has the same shape as a hen's egg. More sensibly, birds deliver their eggs with the small end or diameter presenting through the birth canal. Humans have a similar strategy but sometimes it goes wrong and the fetal head deflexes or, worse still, partially extends on the neck. This creates a bigger cephalic diameter to pass through the maternal pelvis. The two ends of the egg are similar to the suboccipito-bregmatic diameter of a well-flexed vertex presentation and the submento-bregmatic diameter of a face presentation. The long axis of the egg represents the mento-vertical diameter of a brow presentation which is associated with an attitude of partial extension. And so egg-laying birds have need for neither midwives nor obstetricians.

Without OP positions, we wouldn't need obstetricians

Probably the commonest cause of difficulty and delay in labour in the human species is related to malposition, especially occipito-posterior position with a vertex presentation (OP). This is because it takes more work (uterine contractions) for rotation and is often associated with uterine inertia. In addition, it is associated with an attitude of deflection of the fetal head leading to a relatively larger cephalic diameter (occipito-frontal) passing through the pelvis. Moreover, the cervix may dilate in an irregular fashion over the deflexed head leaving a rim of cervix to one side, delaying the progress in the first stage of labour. Some rotate spontaneously to the occipito-anterior position and deliver while others deliver in the direct OP position; but many need obstetric interventions to effect delivery.

Be very sceptical of the 'deflexed OA'

It is a concern when a clinician describes the result of a vaginal assessment for lack of progress as a 'deflexed OA' and the concern is on two counts: first, the combination of a deflexed head and an occipito-anterior position with a vertex presentation do not go together and defy an understanding of the mechanism of labour (unless the pelvis is very capacious and the baby small, in which case there would not be a delay in the labour); secondly, deflexion is most commonly associated with OP and it must be suspected that the clinical assessment has been incorrect.

Similarly, asynclitism, which is lateral flexion of the head, is not observed with OA position and vertex presentations, although severe asynclitism may lead to a parietal presentation but this is usually either anterior or posterior asynclitism. In which case, watch out for cord prolapse in the second stage of labour.

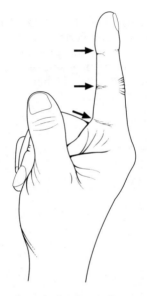

The distance from the introitus to the presenting part
helps determine the mode and type of delivery.

A digital examination will determine station; and the degree of difficulty of the delivery

Should an instrumental delivery be needed it is very important to determine the degree of difficulty. One important assessment is that of station. The station refers to the level of the head in the pelvis but the most important part is the biparietal diameter, which is the widest part of the fetal head. This can be relatively easily assessed with the use of this rule and the index finger.

- One phalanx to the fetal head: generally means the biparietal diameter has passed through the level of the ischial spines (the narrowest part of the pelvis). This is an outlet delivery which even the most inexperienced clinician should be able to perform and successfully deliver the baby.
- Two phalanges to the fetal head: means the biparietal diameter is at or just above the level of the ischial spines. This is a mid-cavity delivery which should be performed by an experienced operator as it may not descend any further.
- Three phalanges to the fetal head: means that the biparietal diameter is at or just above the level of the pelvic inlet and the presenting part may not be engaged. The baby should be delivered by Caesarean section.

Exception

The exception is the very shallow pelvis where the head may almost be visible at the introitus and still not be engaged.

Position and station are determined by palpation; and confirmed by vaginal examination

Assessments in the second stage of labour should not vary for any other time in maternity care. If called to assess why a woman has not delivered despite desperate expulsive maternal efforts the tendency is to don a glove and perform a vaginal examination.

Not so hasty: peruse the partogram, assess the well-being and size of the mother and baby, then perform an abdominal palpation to assess the nature of the contractions, the size of the baby, the position and the degree of engagement of the head, and the attitude, should the head be palpable.

Record the findings. Then perform the vaginal assessment. It then functions as a quality control exercise to confirm what was deduced from the abdominal palpation. Then plan the intervention depending on the previous assessments. Let's not lose our clinical skills.

Syntometrine is a great combination to prevent postpartum haemorrhage

Tonic contraction of the uterus effectively occludes the spiral arteries as they pass through the myometrium. This "living ligature" is essential for survival as the uterine blood flow at term is 500–800 ml/minute. The active management of the third stage as a routine preventive measure is associated with a two-to-threefold reduction in the risk of primary postpartum haemorrhage (PPH).

Physiological management of the third stage has been the choice of some mothers but there is ample evidence to suggest that this choice exposes the mother to increased ($\times 3$) risk of PPH as a consequence of delay in emptying the uterus and blood loss over 1000 ml.[1]

The payoff for using ergometrine-containing oxytocics is a high rate of nausea and vomiting (21–28%) and transient hypertension. Oxytocin alone may be a safe alternative with a more acceptable side-effect profile but may slightly increase the rate of severe postpartum haemorrhage.[2] Carboprost, an analogue of prostaglandin $PGF_{2\alpha}$, is an effective second-line drug for a refractory atonic uterus but must never be administered intravenously.

[1]Prendiville W *et al*. The Bristol third stage trial: "active" vs "physiological" management of the third stage of labour. *BMJ* 1988; **297**: 1295–300.

[2]McDonald SL *et al*. Randomised controlled trial of oxytocin alone versus oxytocin and ergometrine in active management of third stage of labour. *BMJ* 1993; **307**: 1167–71.

Never pull on the cord without a contraction

There are two complications consequent to this most dangerous practice, both of which are avoidable. The first is haemorrhage and shock. The second occurs when the placenta has not separated and uterine inversion follows.

In this event: resuscitate with IV fluids, organise a general anaesthetic, revert the uterus with the hydrostatic method, which requires a large-bore silastic tube, 5–10 litres of saline, and a vaginal pack after the uterus has been manually replaced in the vagina. It is a good idea to wear a plastic apron and do not be surprised how much the vagina distends and how much fluid it requires. After the uterus reverts it must be kept well-contracted, keep the bladder empty, give prophylactic antibiotics, and check the haemoglobin concentration and serum electrolytes for haemodilution.

The reason for induction will be the reason for Caesarean section

This is an old rule which was around in the times before prostaglandins were available and the only option available was a medical and surgical induction (ARM + oxytocin infusion). The obstetrician was then committed to deliver the baby. In other words, the intervention was performed on the basis that the baby had to be delivered. With the advent of cervical ripening agents it has become possible to intervene but without the commitment to deliver the baby. When a medical and surgical induction of labour was unsuccessful, and a Caesarean section was necessary to deliver the baby, then the indication for the induction became the indication for the Caesarean section. In many ways this rule is now not true, but the concept behind it remains good and real, and may serve to reduce unnecessary inductions of labour, or over-intervention in this aspect of pregnancy management.

Induction for post-maturity with a view to deliver the baby after 41 weeks and before 42 completed weeks has been shown to reduce other interventions like Caesarean sections, instrumental deliveries, and adverse outcomes like fetal distress and perinatal morbidity and mortality.[1] It has been calculated that as many as 500 post-term inductions may be necessary to avoid one late unexplained stillbirth. With this level of intervention required to prevent one death it would seem reasonable for clinicians to put serious thought to induction of labour for those women where the odds of unexplained stillbirth may be less favourable, but where evidence to intervene is still lacking.

The clinical situations where it may be wise not to allow mothers to go too far past term and to offer induction of labour include:

- women with diabetes mellitus prior to pregnancy (39 weeks' gestation)
- women with essential hypertension on treatment
- women with undiagnosed antepartum haemorrhage and/or evidence of feto-maternal haemorrhage for whatever reason
- women with a twin pregnancy
- women with less common medical conditions, e.g. renal disease, intrahepatic cholestasis (38 weeks' gestation), systemic lupus erythematosus
- nulliparous woman over 40 years of age

[1] Crowley P. Elective induction at 41+ weeks' gestation. In: Enkin MW, Keirse MJNC, Renfrew MJ, Neilson JP, Crowther C, eds. Pregnancy and Childbirth Module. The Cochrane and Childbirth Database. The Cochrane Collaboration, Issue 2. Oxford: Update Software, 1995.

Use this space to write down your own labour ward rules.

2 Fetal monitoring

Choose which assessment is necessary to monitor the baby

Continuous electronic fetal monitoring during labour with an increased likelihood of fetal decompensation is accepted good practice. Cardiotocography (CTG) is a test or assessment that should be applied to particular clinical situations (see Table 2.1 below). It is not necessary for routine continuous CTGs in all labours and clinicians must be able to justify its use because the assessment may lead to inappropriate interventions.[1] The best method of monitoring the fetus in uncomplicated normal pregnancies is uncertain but intermittent auscultation is a minimum requirement every 15 minutes in the first stage of labour and after each contraction in the second stage.

Table 2.1   Cases in which a continuous CTG should be used.

Maternal	*Fetal*
Hypertension	Prolonged labour
Pre-eclampsia	Augmented labour
Diabetes	Preterm labour
Epilepsy	Infection
Rhesus disease	Meconium stained liquor
Heart disease	Oligohydramnios
Respiratory conditions leading to hypoxia	Audible abnormal heart rate
Renal failure	Intrauterine growth restriction
Renal transplants	Breech presentation
Thyroid disease	Multiple pregnancy
Epidural analgesia (?)	Antepartum haemorrhage
Previous uterine scar	Intrapartum haemorrhage
Inability to auscultate fetal heart (obesity)	Abnormal admission test[2]
Previous fetal loss	

[1]Neilson JP. Cardiotocography during labour. *BMJ* 1993; **306**: 347–8.

[2]Ingemarsson I *et al.* Admission test – a screening test for fetal distress in labor. *Obstet Gynecol* 1986; **68**: 800–6.

To avoid false positives use: CTG + FBS

Any test that has a high false-positive rate, i.e. low specificity, must employ a second-line test to refute false-positives and to reduce inappropriate interventions. This is provided by fetal blood sampling (FBS) which, with a cut-off of pH = 7.20, enables the clinician to classify the CTG as a true or false positive and to act appropriately regardless of the other parameters available on most blood gas analysers. There are some situations that require immediate delivery of the fetus, e.g. prolonged (>9 minutes) fetal bradycardia, cord prolapse, intrapartum abruption, rather than losing time performing an FBS. Decisions concerning suspicious or abnormal CTGs may be made on the assessment of the FBS pH in conjunction with parameters such as the $P\text{CO}_2$ and base excess. In the event of a metabolic acidosis, delivery is indicated but primary respiratory acidosis may be managed conservatively with the correction of any underlying causes like uterine hyperstimulation, epidural complications, and posture-related problems.

Exception

Chorioamnionitis can occasionally confound clinicians and a situation where care is required is in the presence of intrauterine infection. The fetus may respond with a tachycardia which can sometimes become complicated (with decelerations and/or loss of variability) and the development of fetal acidosis in these cases is a late and lethal complication of septicaemia and shock. Therefore, in this situation, the CTG may not be a valid measure of fetal well-being necessitating intervention to protect the fetus. In addition, the fetal blood sampling itself may enhance the risk of septicaemia for the fetus. In this particular clinical situation, local guidelines should be established to deal with the problem but in general the baby should be delivered and passed to the neonatologists for observation, investigation, and antibiotic therapy.

If Caesarean section were required intrauterine swabs for culture must be obtained and high-dose intraoperative and postoperative antibiotics given to protect the mother from septicaemia and wound infection.

Table 2.2 Classification of CTGs in the first stage of labour.

	Baseline Rate	Variability	Decelerations	Accelerations
Normal	110–150 bpm	10–25 bpm	None	Presence of accelerations is reassuring. Not enough evidence to comment on their absence in an otherwise normal trace
Suspicious	100–109 bpm 151–170 bpm	5–9 bpm >25 bpm	Early deceleration Variable deceleration Single prolonged deceleration of up to 3 minutes	None
Pathological	<100 bpm >170 bpm	<5 bpm for >20 min	Late deceleration Prolonged deceleration of >3 minutes	N/A
Pathological	"Sinusoidal" trace: a smooth wave form of 2–5 cycles/min lasting >20 min	None	N/A	N/A

© August 1997, October 1999, Nottingham City Hospital Maternity Unit CTG Interpretation Group.

Table 2.3 Classification of CTGs in the second stage of labour.

Classification	Baseline Rate	Variability	Decelerations	Accelerations
Normal	110–150 bpm If CTG normal, baseline 100–109 bpm or 151–160 bpm is acceptable	10–25 bpm	Early decelerations with rapid recovery	Not enough evidence to comment on their absence in an otherwise normal labour
Suspicious	161–170 bpm 90–99 bpm	5–9 or >25 bpm for 10–20 min	Variable decelerations or any deceleration with slow recovery to baseline after contraction has finished or lasting >2 min	N/A
Pathological	>170 bpm <90 bpm	<5 bpm for 10 min	Late deceleration or bradycardia >3 min	N/A
Pathological	"Sinusoidal" trace: a smooth wave form of 2–5 cycles/min lasting >20 min	None	N/A	N/A

©1997, January 2000, Nottingham City Hospital Maternity Unit CTG Interpretation Group.

It is essential that *all* labour ward staff know the ups and downs of the CTG

Cardiotocography (CTG) records the changes in fetal heart rate. The basic flaw with this approach is that we do not fully understand the fetal physiology which is responsible for the variations observed in the fetal heart rate pattern. However, monitoring the fetal heart is all that is currently available and most monitoring systems are quite robust to cope with the rigours of labour. As a test of fetal well-being it has proven to be sensitive (about 98%) but not particularly specific (60–70%) for fetal acidosis and there is considerable inter- and intra-observer variation with interpretation and classification. In addition, the quality of recordings sometimes confounds its interpretation. As a test it has four independent parameters – base rate, intrinsic variability, accelerations, and decelerations – within the recording, each of which may have a different significance depending on the particular clinical situation. Some of the test parameters may be normal whilst others are abnormal, which adds to the difficulties in interpretation. In the past, abnormal CTGs may have gone unrecognised and led to long delays after the onset of fetal compromise. This was not a defect of the monitoring tool as much as a reflection of poor education and response times of and by birth attendants.

CTGs should be classified according to agreed criteria (see Tables 2.2 and 2.3) as:

- Normal
- Suspicious
- Pathological

In the modern management of labour it is imperative to employ a system CTG education and audit programme to ensure that all the staff have a high standard of CTG interpretation, classification, and necessary actions to prevent intrapartum fetal damage and inappropriate interventions.

Relax the womb to nourish the babe

The uterine artery blood flow to the placenta (500–1000 ml/minute) is severely diminished during uterine contractions and so the fetus has to compensate during uterine diastole. Therefore uterine hyperstimulation can seriously compromise fetal well-being and is a very common complication of the administration of oxytocics for induction or augmentation of labour.

For the mother, the uterine artery is a low priority circulation in the maternal autonomic control of blood pressure and so, when the maternal circulatory system is compromised by haemorrhage, postural supine hypotension, and/or vasodilatory effects of epidural analgesia, the uterine arterial system will constrict and reduce maternal placental blood flow for the fetus.

Similarly, in the fetus with compromised placental function that results in catabolic metabolism and/or a chronic lack of oxygen, there exists a sensitive and powerful autonomic control of blood flow to organs which, if activated, will preferentially supply the fetal brain, adrenal glands, heart, and placenta, at the expense of other vascular beds. This preferential redistribution of blood flow will ultimately contribute to the metabolic acidosis and explains the observation that a severely acidotic baby appears floppy, pale, and shocked with poor peripheral circulation, i.e. pulseless or asphyxiated.

When asked to review a CTG in labour: Stop, look, and listen

The CTG must be interpreted in the context of the clinical situation.

Therefore:

Stop: Assess carefully the situation of the mother, baby, and the labour. Examine the antenatal case notes and the partogram up to that point. Consider how the mother is coping with the labour and how much support she is getting from her partner.

Look: Look at the whole CTG trace to assess any drift in the parameters, especially the base rate. Pull the whole trace out from the machine and examine it from the start. It represents a real-time record of how that baby is responding and coping with the stress of labour.

Listen: Listen to the attendant midwife to consider her/his concerns and observations, especially about the amniotic fluid. Make sure that someone has listened manually to the fetal heart to ensure that what one sees on the recording is what is actually happening.

Double bloods make good records of birth

It is important in this day and age that clinicians provide supporting evidence that they have effected their duty of care to the women and babies under their responsibility correctly.

While there is only a weak relationship between fetal acidosis ($pH < 7 \cdot 11$) and condition at birth and longer-term development, an objective measure like umbilical arterial and venous blood gas analyses will provide information to refute the notion that the cause of disability was related to an intrapartum event.

Double bloods should be obtained in the following circumstances:

- operative deliveries
- previous FBS
- meconium stained liquor

Table 2.4   An example of results from matched fetal umbilical arterial and venous samples in acute respiratory acidosis with impending hypoxia.

	Venous	Normal mean ($\pm$ s.d.)	Arterial	Normal mean ($\pm$ s.d.)
pH	7·23	7·32 (0·07)	6·93	7·26 (0·08)
CO_2	8·22	5·5 (1·18)	17·2	6·0 (1·55)
O_2	5·12	3·85 (0·93)	0·17	2·36 (0·84)
HCO_3 (standardised)	21·0		14·8	
Base excess (blood)	− 3·2	− 6·8 (3·6)	− 9·7	− 6·7 (3·6)

Meconium stained liquor: Assume the worst and hope for the best

Meconium stained liquor (MSL) is the presence of fetal faeces which is sterile and contains bile acids to give the green discoloration. It is observed in 15–20% of term labours, is not necessarily a prerequisite for fetal hypoxia, and may indicate normal physiology. However, it may represent a fetus in distress becoming acidotic and "straining" to get out. Other pathological processes like fetal diarrhoea caused by infection (especially *Listeria monocytogenes*), congenital thyrotoxicosis, and some drugs, may cause MSL.

The grade or thickness of meconium stained amniotic fluid is a function of the amount of liquor present at the time of fetal bowel action. The thicker the meconium the greater the risk of meconium aspiration syndrome. Attempts have been made to grade meconium, e.g. thin and stale green (Grade I), moderate (Grade II), thick and fresh green (Grade III), but this distinction is of little value in clinical practice.

Amnioinfusion with warm isotonic saline in labour has been recently employed to dilute Grade III meconium in an attempt to reduce the risk of meconium aspiration syndrome with some success and perhaps should be considered as a possible therapeutic intervention in labour in the future.

Liquor volume: Take great care with too much or too little

Polyhydramnios may predispose to umbilical cord prolapse and preterm delivery (if it accumulates rapidly). An ultrasound scan prior to rupture of the membranes may detect a cord presentation and avoid acute fetal and obstetric embarrassment. Excess amniotic fluid may also represent some fetal congenital abnormality. After birth a nasogastric tube must be passed to exclude the diagnosis of tracheo-oesophageal fistula and a thorough neonatal examination performed.

Amniotic fluid volume observed during antenatal ultrasound scan assessments correlate with perinatal mortality rates (PNMR):

- 1 cm pool, PNMR = 200/1000 births
- 2 cm pool, PNMR = 50/1000 births
- 3 cm pool, PNMR = 10/1000 births

Therefore if little or no liquor is observed after spontaneous or artificial rupture of the fetal membranes or during labour, the pregnancy should be deemed to be complicated by oligohydramnios and must be monitored carefully throughout the labour.

Another tip: be very careful about rupturing the membranes in the presence of a suspected placental abruption when the fetus is alive, as it may decompress the intrauterine cavity and lead to further rapid separation of the placenta with dire fetal consequences.

3 Operative deliveries

Before any instrumental delivery always consider: FORCEPS

This rule provides a checklist for the operator to consider before delivery.

- **F:** Fully dilated: that is, the second stage of labour, if not, the baby may need to be delivered by Caesarean section.
- **O:** Occiput: that is, the operator must know the position and the station of the fetal head in the maternal pelvis.
- **R:** Ruptured membranes: if not, rupture them and the baby may deliver spontaneously.
- **C:** Contractions: a woman must have contractions to deliver a baby and to prevent postpartum haemorrhage in the third stage.
- **E:** Empty the bladder to protect it, prevent obstruction, and postpartum haemorrhage.
- **P:** Protect the perineum with an episiotomy, with a carefully controlled delivery of the head over the perineum.
- **S:** "Spinal": that is, an adequate form of local or regional analgesia.

Choose your instrument and location, and then try well, once

The choice of instrument will depend on the prevailing conditions and the experience and training of the operator. This rule states that there is no place for multiple attempts at instrumental delivery. The operator must assess the degree of difficulty and give good consideration to the location for the attempted delivery. For rotational and some mid-cavity non-rotational deliveries it may be best to perform in a location where there is easy and quick access to facilities to perform a Caesarean section should the attempt be unsuccessful.

Exception

The possible exceptions include: when the ventouse becomes detached at the pelvic outlet; or when the operator has a preference for straight traction forceps following rotation.

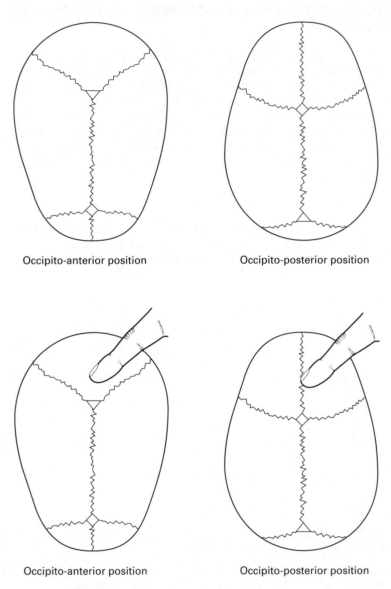

Occipito-anterior position

Occipito-posterior position

Occipito-anterior position

Occipito-posterior position

Feeling for the sutres to determine the position.

The use of the ventouse is not an excuse for not determining fetal position

This rule states the obvious. Should the position prove too difficult to determine, a more experienced operator should be called upon to give a second opinion. If the position cannot be determined because of too much caput and moulding the labour may well be obstructed and instrumental delivery contraindicated. Moreover, the correct positioning of the ventouse cap on the flexion point of the fetal head requires an appreciation of fetal position and degree of flexion. The key to the determination of the fetal position rests with the identification of the sagittal suture followed by the parieto-parietal suture (anterior fontanelle) or confirmation of its absence (posterior fontanelle). This is best achieved by pressing one's index finger and nail from the fronto-parietal sutures to feel for the midline suture or between the occipito-parietal sutures where no midline suture is detected.

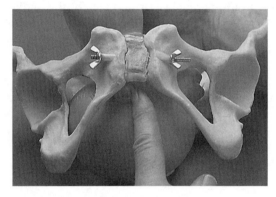

Feeling for the fetal ear.

Feel for the ear, and all will be clear

Another useful tip is to attempt to confirm the fetal position by feeling for the fetal ear. When it can be reached it means that there is a reasonable amount of space in the maternal pelvis and helps in the determination of the station as the ear is close to the biparietal diameter. The position can be confirmed by flipping the finger backwards and forwards to determine the direction in which the ear is positioned.

For malpositions, try a digital rotation first

In these days of epidural analgesia, delay in the second stage is common and often associated with a malposition. When called to assess the situation it is very helpful to be able to assess how tight the fit is with the fetal head and the maternal pelvis.

With a lateral position it is worth trying to rotate the fetal head to the occipito-anterior position by applying a rotational force with the index finger on the appropriate occipito-parietal suture with a contraction aided by maternal expulsive effort. It is important not to push upwards as the head may be disengaged.

This will serve two purposes: it may result in a spontaneous delivery without the need of obstetrical instrumentation or convert a rotational delivery into a straight forceps; with no rotation it will tell the operator that some form of rotational delivery will be necessary and there is a snug or tight fit. For those experienced with rotational forceps it is often easier to apply the forceps blades in the direct occipito-posterior position and so right or left occipito-posterior positions may be rotated back to the direct occipito-posterior position before direct application of the rotational forceps.

Rest the bladder and it will give you peace

It is important to remember to rest the bladder after an instrumental delivery, especially when associated with the use of epidural analgesia. A urinary catheter left on free drainage until the following morning will not increase the risk of urinary tract infection and will avoid urinary retention, either recognised or unrecognised. It is also important to help prevent delayed postpartum haemorrhage.

This rule could also be applied to postoperative management of Caesarean section and manual removal of the placenta.

Incise the lower segment 1 cm below the peritoneal reflection

Caesarean sections in the second stage of labour can be difficult, especially when the presenting part is the breech, and the lower segment is prone to tear and bleed. To prevent performing an unplanned colporrhaphy, define the level where the peritoneum inserts into the upper segment of the myometrium (it is often more superior than one thinks!) and make the uterine incision 1 cm below this point.

Secure the angles first and all will go well

This rule encourages the surgeon to define the uterine angles on both sides before proceeding to suture the first and haemostatic layer with a continuous suture. Most surgeons close the uterine muscle with two layers (although one may suffice), the aim of the second being to invert the first ischaemic layer into the uterine cavity. Any debris or blood can then pass out of the uterus rather than forming a collection.

Following this rule, the surgeon does not have to suture laterally from the marked angles and thus avoids the perils of the broad ligaments and the uterine veins therein or bowel behind. In addition, the surgeon knows that no part of the uterine wall has been left unsecured.

For inferior angle tears directed towards the cervix the lower end should be defined and sutured in one layer upwards towards the uterine incision and then tied off. Tears of this type are a consequence of the surgeon not disimpacting the fetal head in the midline with a tendency to pull the head towards the surgeon thus tearing the opposite side. Always try to disimpact the head upward in the maternal midline to avoid trouble.

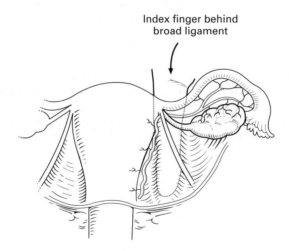

Index finger behind
broad ligament

To stop bleeding and to determine the lateral angle of the
uterine incision.

Bleeding at the angle: Put your finger behind the broad ligament

This rule follows on from the previous one. By placing an index finger behind the broad ligament the bleeding will stop and enable the surgeon to identify the site of haemorrhage and to place sutures in the correct position and avoid misplacement in the broad ligament with its potentially serious complications.

Check posteriorly for
occult uterine trauma

Check the posterior aspect of the uterus.

Always look at the posterior uterine wall

The rule is really a safety check after difficult operations and with continuous haemorrhage. Inspection of the posterior uterine wall may well reveal an extended lower segment uterine tear which had not previously been identified. It is an unusual surgical complication but one well worth remembering when the going gets tough and may just prevent a Caesarean hysterectomy.

If this operation needs to be performed, it is essential that the vaginal vault is very well sutured; interrupted sutures with no gaps between, followed by insertion of a vaginal drain, are to be recommended.

Never attempt a myomectomy at Caesarean section

Fibroids have an extensive blood supply, especially in pregnancy, and so it is an important rule to follow not to be tempted to perform a myomectomy at Caesarean section, to avoid excessive haemorrhage. If the lower uterine segment is covered with fibroids, an upper uterine incision should be performed. In addition, it is an unnecessary procedure as the fibroids will shrink rapidly in the puerperium, especially if the mother should breast feed.

Damaged bowel: Cover up then clean up

In the event of inadvertent damage to the bowel, especially on entering the peritoneal cavity during a Caesarean section, the surgeon should not panic but take a dry swab and cover up the wound to minimise peritoneal spillage and contamination. Continue the Caesarean section and deliver the baby and complete the procedure. Then return to the bowel damage and correct it using a double layer closure technique. Wash out the peritoneal cavity well with an aqueous antiseptic solution, give parenteral antibiotics (loading dose of gentamicin and metronidazole), and close the abdomen.

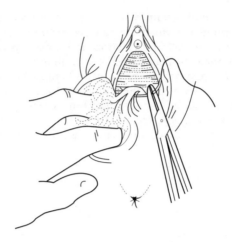

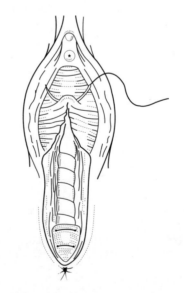

A knot at the top of the vaginal incision is essential to stop heamorrhage.

A knot at the top will stop the lot

When suturing a vaginal laceration it is essential to secure the whole of the vaginal wall, especially the superior aspect of the trauma. When difficulty is experienced try inserting a suture and using this to apply traction to pull the vagina down into the operator's view and to provide access to insert another suture above the traction suture.

Good light, good access, good assistance, and good technique

Some vaginal lacerations can extend to the upper third and vault where access can be difficult and the operator needs optimal exposure and assistance to obtain haemostasis. When the conditions are not suitable to achieve this aim the surgeon must insist on: good light to visualise the bleeding points, good assistance to gain good access to enable good surgical technique to procure a good result.

Pressure stops bleeding

When vaginal or uterine bleeding is persistent despite the surgeon's best attempts it is important not to panic and to re-consider the situation. To do this the surgeon needs some time and time can be gained by simply applying manual pressure to the bleeding vagina, or bimanual compression to the uterus.

This will allow the surgeon to regain composure and to:

- call for assistance
- get some blood cross-matched and perform clotting studies
- assess the blood loss and
- resuscitate the patient as required.

Often, to the great relief of the surgeon, the pressure itself achieves haemostasis. Catheterise the urinary bladder, leave the bladder to drain continuously, transfuse liberally and correct any coagulopathy, give prophylactic antibiotics, and ensure that the uterus remains well-contracted.

When a pack is left in the vagina, be careful

Try to resist the temptation to leave a vaginal pack *in situ* for two good reasons:

- it will act as a nidus of infection, and
- it may obscure and delay the diagnosis of recurrent haemorrhage which may lead to shock, consumption coagulopathy, renal failure, and death.

Should a pack be left, it must be removed the next morning and careful patient observations are essential during this time.

Always follow up the mother and baby after an operative delivery

It is a very important aspect of care to review the outcome of the operative deliveries and to make sure there are no complications. Not only does it give the operator an opportunity to assess quality assurance but enables a debriefing with the mother to make sure she understands why she required an operative intervention and enables the operator to answer any questions.

Should the baby be admitted to the Neonatal Unit it is mandatory for obstetricians to monitor the progress and to keep in touch with the outcome in the long term. A good obstetrician is always seen on the Neonatal Unit.

Use this space to write down your own labour ward rules.

4 Complex deliveries

There is no subject more controversial than breech deliveries

This rule will hold until controlled trials provide clinicians with data on an effective approach. The subject remains controversial because breech presentations are infrequent and are not infrequently associated with other conditions that impact on perinatal outcome, notably: preterm labour, multiple pregnancies, placenta praevia, umbilical cord complications, and congenital abnormalities. Routine elective Caesarean section is not necessarily the answer as it does not appear to prevent long-term handicap in the babies.[1] These issues can be summed up in the dilemma of breech deliveries (Rule 4.2).

Recent data

The Multicentre Term Breech Trial[2] has provided randomised controlled data to indicate that planned Caesarean section can reduce the overall risk of perinatal death for term complete or frank breeches by 75% (Relative risk=0.23; CI 0.07–0.8).

ong-term outcome by method of delivery of fetuses in breech
population-based follow-up. *BMJ* 1996; **312**: 1451–3.
nned Caesarean section versus planned vaginal birth for breech
randomised multicentre trial. *Lancet* 2000; **356**: 1368–9.

The breech dilemma: Dead easy, Easy dead

This may seem a rather harsh rule but it depicts the dilemma with labour when the presenting part is the breech, which confers risk independent of the mode of delivery. Often breech deliveries can be quick and easy and very satisfying for all involved and so this rule should evoke confidence while careful assessment should alert the clinician to the possible need for an early intervention.

Spontaneous breech delivery relies on pushing forces from the mother rather than traction from birth attendants. Assisted breech delivery is supposed to enable control of the baby to prevent delay and malposition but risks trauma and alteration in fetal attitude. Attempts to avoid the breech dilemma have led to the use of external cephalic version at term or early labour. It has been shown to be beneficial in reducing intervention in the form of a subsequent Caesarean section (odds ratio = $0 \cdot 42$, 95% confidence interval $0 \cdot 29$ to $0 \cdot 62$) without any increased risk to the fetus.

Delivery of the unmoulded head is a part of the breech problem

When the presenting part is a breech the attitude can be flexed (flexed at the knees and the hips, **complete**) or extended (extended at the knees and flexed at the hips, **frank**). The presenting part may be breech but the presentation foot/feet, commonly called a footling breech (extended at the knees and the hips), all are classified as malpresentations.

The breech is smaller than the head and it is the delivery of the unmoulded fetal head which creates the potential for problems and perinatal morbidity and mortality and is associated with too slow or too rapid delivery of the head.

Delay with the delivery of the fetal head can be caused by relative cephalo-pelvic disproportion; extended attitude of the head when the mentum is caught on the sacral promontory, malposition (occipito-posterior), or absolute cephalo-pelvic disproportion. The cervix must be fully taken up into the lower segment of the uterus to avoid causing delay in the second stage. The incompletely dilated cervix is the major problem, especially with the preterm and footling breeches, as the presenting part may pass through the partially dilated cervix and give the mother an uncontrollable urge to push. However, the unmoulded head will not descend past the cervix and result in delay in delivery of the head, cord compression, asphyxia, and probably fetal trauma from uncontrolled efforts to deliver the baby.

Obviously this situation is best avoided by:

- considering Caesarean section for all footling breeches
- the use of epidural analgesia to prevent premature expulsive maternal effort, especially in multiparous women
- ensure full dilatation of the cervix by waiting for descent of the breech on to the perineum before pushing commences
- progress in the first stage of labour should be exemplary

If one applies traction during a breech delivery one must understand the consequences

It has often been said that one should never pull on the breech during an assisted breech delivery. This may be a good rule for those who do not have any understanding of the consequences of fetal traction but may lead to delay in completion of the delivery and prolonged cord compression.

It is a simple law of physics: "To every action there is an equal and opposite reaction" and so the consequences of traction on the baby with a breech presentation is the conversion of the baby's attitude from flexion to extension of the arms and neck. If one understands these reactions one is in a position to predict the need to bring down the extended arms and then to flex the head on the neck, usually with the index finger in the fetal mouth, to effect a safe delivery when traction was necessary. However, the earlier in the delivery one applies traction to the baby and the more manipulation required, the greater the risk of fetal trauma and damage.

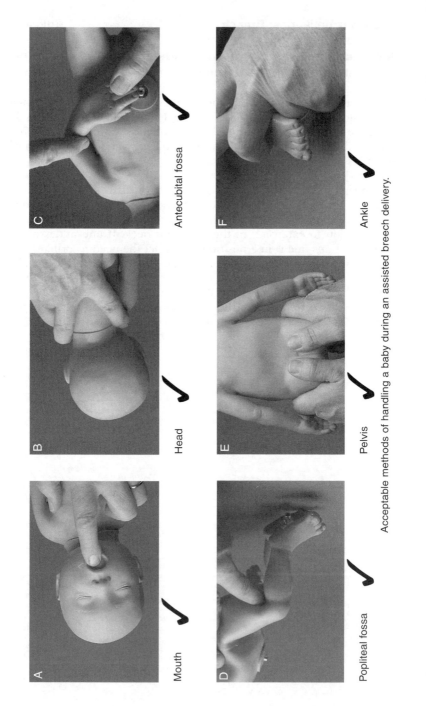

Mouth

Head

Antecubital fossa

Popliteal fossa

Pelvis

Ankle

Acceptable methods of handling a baby during an assisted breech delivery.

The breech baby must be handled carefully with correct and acceptable manipulations

Breech deliveries, either at Caesarean section or vaginal delivery, must not become a 'no-holds-barred' wrestling match or a test of strength between the baby and the deliverer, as there is no doubt that the attendant is stronger than the baby and trauma and fetal damage will be a predictable consequence. The fact is that there are a finite number of acceptable places to hold the baby to effect safe delivery and an infinite number of unacceptable holds.

Correct and acceptable fetal manipulations

- Mouth (traction, rotation, and to flex neck)
- Head (traction, forceps to after-coming head)
- Antecubital fossa (to flex elbow)
- Popliteal fossa (to flex knee)
- Pelvis (traction and rotation)
- Ankle (traction)

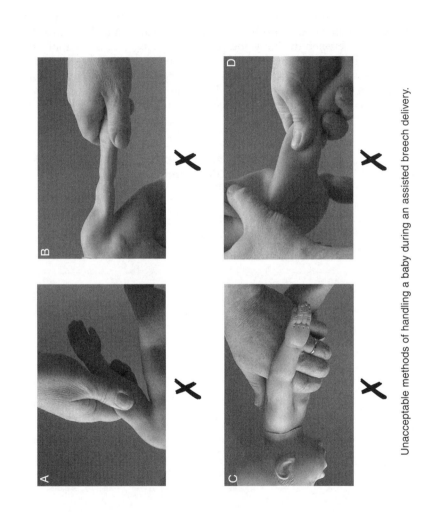

Unacceptable methods of handling a baby during an assisted breech delivery.

Incorrect and unacceptable fetal manipulations

Any other hold may result in bruising and fractures or visceral and nerve damage. In addition, one should always avoid applying traction on the fetal wrist/hand as it will convert the presentation into a shoulder and obstruct the delivery, especially at Caesarean section. Always try to convert deliveries to breech in the event of a transverse lie by applying traction to the fetal foot; should a hand be inadvertently grasped it should be immediately released and replaced into the uterus and a foot sought.

Exception

The only acceptable time to apply traction to a hand is in a severe shoulder dystocia in an attempt to deliver a posterior shoulder (see later).

Flat at birth, call the paediatrician first

After a vaginal breech delivery the baby may be shocked and stunned by the rapid delivery of the fetal head through the pelvis and following a degree of umbilical cord compression. It is important to keep the baby warm by wrapping the delivered legs and trunk with a dry towel. Most important for the baby is to have an experienced, well-trained person present at the delivery dedicated solely for the assessment and resuscitation of the baby as required.

Be selective and be careful

When external cephalic version is inappropriate or unsuccessful it is essential to select women with breech presentations who should not be considered for vaginal delivery:

- uterine scar
- large baby
- small pelvis
- intrauterine growth restriction
- hyperextension of the fetal head
- placenta praevia
- maternal medical illnesses
- maternal desire to avoid vaginal delivery

These women should be delivered by elective Caesarean section.

Recourse to Caesarean section is to be recommended when progress in labour is not satisfactory, although augmentation with oxytocics may be justified in certain selected cases. Continuous fetal monitoring should be employed. The incidence of asphyxial episodes decreases with increasing birthweight but the incidence of neonatal trauma increases with increasing birthweight and there probably is an optimal fetal weight for vaginal delivery from about 2500 g to 3800 g.

There are no conclusive data on breech presentation in preterm labour but the aim of the obstetrician should be to deliver the baby in the best possible condition for subsequent neonatal care. The outcome for very low birthweight infants is related to prematurity rather than mode of delivery. Footling breech deliveries are often complicated by cord compression and/or prolapse, premature maternal expulsive efforts, and incomplete dilatation of the cervix and should be delivered by Caesarean section.

Twin labour must aim to: Secure a safe delivery of the second twin and prevent primary postpartum haemorrhage

The management of twin labour must be well controlled, with special attention in the second and third stages. This rule states the two added risks for twin labour above and beyond the singleton labour. Both twins must be monitored adequately as the second twin is at risk of umbilical cord and placental mishaps predisposing it to hypoxia, especially in the second stage of labour, and over-manipulation which may lead to fetal trauma. As a result of over-distension of the uterus the third stage must be managed aggressively to prevent primary postpartum haemorrhage. Knowledge of the current maternal haemoglobin is essential and blood should be cross-matched in readiness.

Be sure the labour has really progressed to the second stage

To secure a safe delivery of the second twin the attendant must be absolutely confident that the cervix is fully taken up into the lower segment. This will help if intrauterine manipulations are necessary. A thorough vaginal assessment to confirm full cervical dilatation is essential. If there is any doubt a reassessment one hour later should be sufficient. Active second stage pushing should only commence once the presenting part of twin one has descended on to the pelvic floor. Epidural analgesia can be very helpful for the attendant in the management of both the second and third stage to achieve the above-mentioned aim.

The active second stage is usually short, if not, trouble may be in store

The active second stage should be short because twin babies are smaller than singletons. If delay is experienced then suspicions should be raised and a full reassessment should occur. The following must be considered:

- locked twins
- malposition
- malpresentation (especially brow)

The labour must not be permitted to continue without the anticipated good progress. Be prepared when an instrumental delivery is required to deliver the first twin, especially in a multiparous woman.

Success with the second twin is all in the timing

This rule emphasises the importance of the timing of interventions: the rupture of the membranes and re-establishing effective uterine contractions to successfully deliver the second twin. The lie must be corrected to longitudinal and the membranes ruptured only when the presenting part is engaged in the pelvis.

In the case of a footling or complete breech, the foot may be grasped through the membranes to expedite the delivery as soon as the membranes are ruptured. Intravenous oxytocin infusion should be initiated after delivery of the first twin and continued after the third stage has been completed.

With preterm twins one must aim to prevent spastic diplegia in the first and cerebral palsy and quadriplegia in the second

This rule suggests that the risk of preterm delivery with twin delivery is the classic cerebral damage associated with prematurity observed in the first twin and combined damage of prematurity and hypoxic ischaemic encephalopathy in the second.

Preterm labour and delivery is common in multiple pregnancies and yet there is no good data to determine the optimal mode of delivery for preterm twins. Issues to be considered in the decision-making process should include:

- gestation and neonatal resources
- zygosity and "amnionicity"
- discordant growth between twins
- presentation of both twins
- ability to monitor both twins
- pregnancy problems: pre-eclampsia, antepartum haemorrhage
- cervical dilatation on presentation
- experience of birth attendants
- maternal age and previous fertility
- maternal wishes

However, the aim must be to endeavour to deliver the babies in the best possible condition for the neonatologist and often Caesarean section will fulfil that aim. Vaginal delivery may be appropriate when women present in the second stage of labour or when fetal survival is unlikely because of the severe prematurity.

Maternal posture may be the only problem

While shoulder dystocia is the ultimate obstetric emergency, many minor difficulties with the delivery of the shoulders may be overcome by obtaining access to allow correct downward traction (not excessive) to deliver the anterior shoulder under the sub-pubic arch. This can often be quickly achieved by rolling the woman to the left lateral position or to place the woman in the lithotomy position.

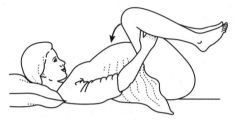

McRobert's manoeuvre
maternal hip flexion and abduction

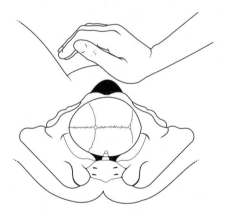

Interventions to resolve shoulder dystocia.

Push don't pull, abduct, rotate, and pray

Should the delivery not be affected with a change in maternal posture it is important to:

- Stop the traction
- Do not panic and call for help – experienced midwives and obstetricians, anaesthetic and paediatric staff
- Apply firm flexion and abduction of the maternal thighs to increase the pelvic inlet
- Apply suprapubic (not fundal) pressure to the anterior shoulder to rotate to the transverse diameter and under the symphysis pubis
- Perform an episiotomy to increase access posteriorly

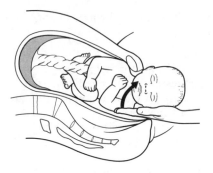

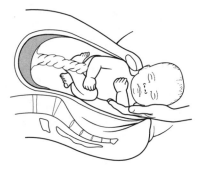

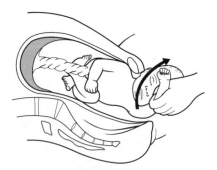

Interventions to resolve a shoulder dystocia.

Should these external measures be unsuccessful, internal manipulations are required with prayer and trepidation:

- Rotation of the posterior shoulder anteriorly under the sub-pubic arch with a corkscrew action
- Attempt to deliver the posterior arm by pushing it posteriorly in the antecubital fossa
- Symphisiotomy
- Clavicular osteotomy
- Replace the fetal head in the vagina and perform a Caesarean section

Always describe in detail the degree of dystocia

It is imperative that the delivery and manoeuvres required to effect the delivery are carefully recorded by all present. This will help in the planning of future deliveries and provide sound medicolegal defence for what is the ultimate unpredictable obstetric emergency.

An umbilical cord blood gas analysis should be obtained after the delivery. The degree of difficulty will be reflected in the amount of damage suffered by the baby, which should also be recorded objectively.

5   Obstetric haemorrhage and shock

Shock in obstetrics is shocking obstetrics

The essence of this rule is that shock as a consequence of haemorrhage should be avoided by a combination of prediction and prevention and rapid response and resuscitation in unexpected haemorrhage. It implies that if shock occurs there has been some oversight in the case assessment. While this is not always the case, substantial haemorrhage and maternal shock should necessitate a thorough case review, possibly through an incident reporting system.

APH + Breech = Placenta praevia until proven otherwise

This is a rule which comes from before the days of ultrasound scanning but the advent of ultrasound imaging does not detract from its essential nature. Scans can be wrong, false negatives are a reality, especially with a posterior placenta. It is an unwise clinician who puts all his/her faith in one scan report when the clinical situation is crying out the answer. A transverse or oblique lie should evoke the same clinical response. In short, assume placenta praevia: cross-match and transfuse if necessary, monitor mother and baby and exclude placenta praevia, deliver if necessary.

Blood between maternal toes is serious blood loss indeed

Accurate assessment of blood loss in obstetrics is always difficult but never more difficult when the woman has arrived in the labour ward from home with heavy vaginal bleeding (usually painless). In addition, young fit women may not appear compromised or shocked by the blood loss because they may compensate for acute blood loss by increasing cardiac output (CO) and maintaining blood pressure (BP) through an increase in stroke volume (SV) rather than heart rate (HR) together with peripheral vasoconstriction or resistance (PR). Remember:

$$CO = HR \times SV; \text{ and } BP = CO \times PR$$

When vaginal blood loss occurs at home and runs down the victim's legs, there appears to be a tendency to wipe up the blood without paying due attention to the feet and toes. Therefore, blood between the toes, which themselves are pale from vasoconstriction, is a tell-tale sign of serious large blood loss and appropriate action is required before the woman decompensates and becomes shocked.

There are three questions to be answered about acute antenatal vaginal haemorrhage

In the event of acute antenatal vaginal haemorrhage the registrar will rightly notify more experienced staff and ask for assistance. To assess if the registrar has the situation under control only three questions need to be asked:

- What is the woman's haemoglobin concentration?
- How much blood has been cross-matched?
- What kind of anaesthetic has been proposed by the anaesthetist?

Should the response be a rustling of papers to find the haemoglobin result; and/or there has been less than four units cross-matched; and/or the anaesthetist has not been contacted or has suggested a regional anaesthetic in a potentially compromised patient, this means that the situation on the labour ward may well be out of control and necessitates a rapid journey to the ward to set things right. So the attendant obstetrician must know the haemoglobin, ensure an adequate cross-match ("four and more") and commence transfusion, and contact the anaesthetist with a view to a general anaesthetic to deliver the baby and stop the haemorrhage.

Exceptions

Some anaesthetists may take exception to this statement but it really implies good communication between obstetric and anaesthetic staff with the aim to avoid profound shock as a consequence of regional anaesthesia and unrecognised cardiovascular compensation. The same may be applied to postpartum haemorrhage.

A lethal abruption: Keep four or more pints of blood at the ready at all times

Fortunately we do not see as many lethal abruptions which lead to sudden intrauterine death, but when it does occur the uterus fills up with blood clot, possibly without much vaginal bleeding. This can trick the inexperienced attendant and the reality is that maternal blood loss is much greater than expected. Moreover, the intrauterine clot contains a large proportion of the woman's total platelets and clotting factors which leads to a consumptive coagulopathy.

Therefore, transfuse freely, keep a reserve of cross-matched blood available for use, monitor clotting often, do not forget the Kleihauer test for iso-immunisation in Rhesus negative women – and remember the next rule.

Always ask about the abruption: 'What's the haemoglobin concentration?'

Essential to the management of the woman with an abruption is a regular reassessment of the haemoglobin concentration, hourly if necessary. To avoid anaemia is paramount. Deliver the baby, placenta, and intrauterine clot (which at times can be bigger than the baby!) as soon as reasonably possible by the safest route. Avoid postpartum haemorrhage (see below). Be in close contact with the blood laboratory and perhaps a specialist haematologist, should replacement of blood products or platelets be necessary.

The storm can be weathered by keeping the mother well-transfused. Once the products of conception have been expelled the blood disorders will settle. Monitor urine output and renal function; as acute renal impairment may be a complication of severe abruption.

Pale and floppy at birth, milk the cord for all its worth

Just occasionally a baby can become anaemic and distressed by virtue of a haemorrhage into the maternal circulation, a so-called feto-maternal or transplacental haemorrhage or rupture of a vasa praevia. The astute clinician will recognise this at the delivery of a pale and floppy infant and promptly transfuse the baby with the blood remaining in the placental circulation (milking the cord) before severing the umbilical cord, thus increasing the fetal circulating blood volume. This prompt response may be life-saving. However, this practice is not to be recommended otherwise, although there are data to suggest that preterm babies may benefit from the gravitational effect of being held below the level of the placenta prior to cutting the umbilical cord.[1]

---

[1] Kinmonds S *et al.* Umbilical cord clamping and preterm infants: a randomised trial. *BMJ* 1993; **306**: 172–5.

APH = PPH

Be prepared and be active: when a woman has suffered an antepartum haemorrhage she is at increased risk of a postpartum haemorrhage. This is particularly true for uterine abruptions large and small. It is advisable for experienced medical staff to be present at the delivery following lethal abruption to oversee the administration of the oxytocic drugs, fluids, and blood, as necessary.

Prevention of postpartum haemorrhage by rapid delivery of the placenta membranes and blood clot is essential in these compromised women. There is no need to wait for placental separation, the abruption has seen to that. Intravenous oxytocics is the method of choice to avoid muscle haematoma formation in the presence of a coagulopathy and where there is reduced peripheral circulation, say: 5 units oxytocin + 500 micrograms ergometrine diluted in 20 ml normal saline titrated slowly according to situation, followed by an infusion of high-strength oxytocin as an infusion (say: 40 units in 500 ml normal saline over 2–4 hours). Uterine bleeding, even with thrombocytopenia and coagulopathy, will be prevented by obtaining a good tonic uterine contraction.

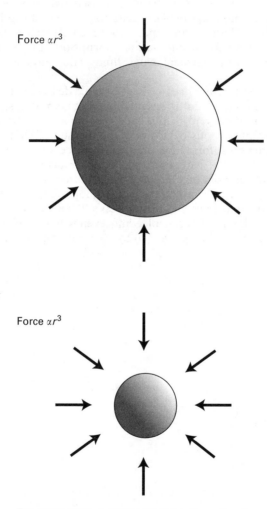

The uterus is like a sphere: the larger the radius, the more the force required to compress it.

The laws of the uterus are elementary physics of a sphere

Everyone knows that uterine contraction after birth is an essential component of the prevention of haemorrhage as the branches of the uterine arteries are twisted and kinked between the interdigitating contracted muscle fibres of the uterus. What is not appreciated is an understanding of the relationship between the forces required to compress a spherical object and the radius of that sphere: compression force α r^3. In other words, in order to compress a uterus to prevent bleeding from the arteries, the force required will be much greater the larger the uterus (r). That is why women with large babies, polyhydramnios, multiple pregnancies etc., etc., will be at greater risk of primary postpartum haemorrhage unless the proper interventions are planned and performed to prevent it. More importantly, this is why it is so essential that the uterus is completely emptied of products of conception and blood clot after birth. And so – remember the next rule.

When in doubt, feel about

When there is doubt about the completeness of the placenta after birth, serious consideration should be given to a manual exploration of the uterine cavity under the appropriate analgesia. It is better to exclude the diagnosis of retained placental parts than to suffer the consequences of serious reactive postpartum haemorrhage. The problem, of course, is that the inspection of the placenta and membranes at the completion of the third stage of labour is a poor test, with low sensitivity and specificity. The answer is to make one's own assessment and in these days of epidural analgesia, it should not be too difficult to arrange with the anaesthetist to quickly and efficiently explore the uterine cavity and remove the offending material or refute the diagnosis.

If there are doubts about a retained placental cotyledon with ongoing vaginal haemorrhage then the intervention is essential and should be expedited. Following that, adminster prophylactic antibiotics and – remember the next rule.

Keep the bladder empty to help the uterus stop bleeding

Perhaps it would be more accurate to write this rule in the negative: "If one does not catheterise the urinary bladder the uterus may bleed." Obviously the uterus is not a true sphere and another part of uterine tonic contractility after birth is anteflexion on itself. To enhance this anteflexion it is advised to keep the bladder empty by an indwelling urinary catheter on free drainage until the next morning (or for 24 hours); but for no longer, as urinary infection may complicate the case.

Once a PPH, always a PPH

This rule particularly refers to uterine atony. Antenatal assessments should have detected this as a problem in labour and the labour ward staff alerted accordingly. Failure to do so would represent a serious oversight.

Once aware of the potential problem, preventative action can be taken; IV access, active management of the third stage, oxytocics, full blood count and group, and save serum for potential cross-match.

Any woman who requires resuscitation after birth needs blood

This follows on from previous rules that women who decompensate and become shocked have lost so much blood that cardiovascular reserve is exhausted. Many women do not want blood transfusions but in this case they often need a blood transfusion. The tendency not to transfuse leads to severe anaemia and its consequences and may be dangerous in the event of secondary postpartum haemorrhage.

Exception

The possible exception to this rule is when a woman has epidural analgesia which has negated the woman's autonomic compensatory capacity.

Use this space to write down your own labour ward rules.

6   Infection

Hand washing is the most effective method of infection prevention

Ignaz Phillip Semmelweis (1818–65) was a Hungarian obstetrician who pioneered asepsis in childbirth. Before the development of the aseptic techniques many women died from ascending infection or puerperal fever. Since the advent of antibiotics, treatment has become available and death from maternal infections are now rare, but not eradicated. The concern will come when the vaginal commensal micro-organisms become more virulent and resistant to commonly used antibiotics. Infections are still with us and remain a threat to child-bearing women and their children; vigilance by maternity workers is essential: always wash your hands between patients.

When dealing with matters concerned with infection consider the Infection Formula

What then are the variables which determine whether sepsis will or will not occur in any one individual, recognising that all child-bearing women are at risk?

Consider the following "Infection Formula":

$$\text{Sepsis} \propto \frac{\text{Type} \times \text{Virulence} \times \text{Load} \times \text{Resistance} \times \text{Site of micro-organisms}}{\text{Host defence}}$$

The following are a few common situations where the Infection Formula can be applied.

Anaerobes like *Bacteroides*, *peptostreptococci* and *Haemophilus gardnerinella* are commensal in the vagina but in a condition like bacterial vaginosis, which is associated with a large load of anaerobes, and, in the right conditions, for example retained intrauterine products of conception, transcervical spread would lead to postnatal endometritis. Most of these anaerobes have already developed penicillin resistance and antibiotics like metronidazole, clindamycin, and the β-lactamase inhibitors clavulanate and tazobactam are necessary. One factor in favour of the host is that the uterus tends to contain intrauterine infection for some time before it is disseminated throughout the body, more so than, say, the urinary tract with organisms like *E. coli*, *Klebsiella* and *Proteus* species.

The enteropharyngeal group include *E. coli*, *Streptococcus faecalis*, *β-haemolytic streptococcus* and *Streptococcus viridans*. All can infect the upper genital tract given the opportunity. Group B *streptococcus* is vaginal commensal (15–30% of women depending on where one lives) and can overgrow and be detected in urine culture, reflecting large lower genital tract carriage. It remains sensitive to penicillin but virulent strains can produce rapid fetal, neonatal, and maternal demise.

Herpes simplex II lower genital tract infection may lead to vertical infection and cause neonatal encephalitis. Many women with recurrent disease shed the virus continually. Fortunately, immunity in these women is passed on to the fetus enhancing host defence and the infants are only at risk if there is a large viral load or the mother's immunity has been obtunded. Neonatal protection can be afforded to women with primary infections by Caesarean section avoiding or reducing exposure.

Insulin-dependent diabetics have reduced host defence and so need antibiotics to prevent infection, especially after Caesarean sections.

In septic shock give them the lot

Septicaemia and septic shock require urgent treatment of hypotension with IV colloids or plasma expanders until the antibiotics are effective. Monitor the blood pressure, oxygen saturation (with pulse oximetry), and urine output. Consult with the obstetric anaesthetist as sometimes intensive care is required with cardiovascular and respiratory support.

Septic shock is most commonly the consequence of virulent strains of urinary or enteropharyngeal micro-organisms which produce endotoxins (especially *E. coli* and Group A and B *streptococci*). The patient must be treated with high-dose penicillin-based antibiotics (unless allergy exists), e.g. penicillin G 2·4 g IV 4-hourly or ampicillin 2 g IV stat and thence 1g IV 4-hourly; metronidazole 500 mg IV or rectally (1 g) is mandatory for the opportunistic anaerobes and an aminoglycoside (gentamicin or vancomycin) for the enteropaths, until the culture results are available with specific sensitivities.

Meta-analysis data has suggested that single daily dose regimes for the aminoglycosides are as effective as multiple daily dose regimes; the regimen is less nephrotoxic, no greater risk of ototoxicity, and is more convenient and cheaper.[1] The quinolones (e.g. ciprofloxacin) are more expensive but give good cover for the pharyngeal streptococci and may be useful for women with penicillin allergy.

For women with a rapid sinus tachycardia (>140 b/m) consideration should be given to the possibility of *Clostridia welshii* infection.

---

[1]Barza M *et al*. Single or multiple doses of aminoglycosides: a meta-analysis. *BMJ* 1996; **312**: 338–45.

Consider carefully the antibiotic therapy: Not just 'Ceph & Met'

Clinicians who prescribe intravenous cephalosporins and metronidazole for serious infections often err when the patient is converted to oral medications. The cefuroxime/cephataxime is converted to oral cephradine and all is lost. Cephradine has poor tissue penetration and is not effective in deep-tissue infection. It is rapidly excreted by the kidneys and is only good in obstetric urine infections, and that's about it. The trouble is there is no good oral equivalent for third generation cephalosporins. Check the culture results and consider a 5-day parenteral course to cure the patient.

In addition, co-amoxiclav (1 g amoxycillin and 200 mg clavulanic acid) 8-hourly IV for severe infections is probably not as effective as other regimens mentioned above: not enough penicillin, poor tissue penetration, and shorter half-life of clavulanate. That is not to say that this combination is not very useful for urinary tract infections, minor cases of puerperal endometritis, and prophylaxis at Caesarean section (proven value in emergency procedures).

Below 25, Chlamydia is alive

Chlamydial cervicitis is common in the young and can have serious consequences for both the mother and baby. It can cause vaginal discharge and recurrent small antepartum haemorrhages. Swab the cervix for at least 10 seconds (this intracellular obligate infects the transformation zone and columnar cell of the endocervix) and treat with erythromycin 500 mg QID for two weeks.

Another macrolide antibiotic, azythromycin 1g stat orally, is very effective and compliance can be observed, although there is no licence for its use in pregnancy.

Remember that proof of cure and contact tracing are integral parts of treating and curing women and their partners of this sexually transmitted infection. Screening the young population is probably of no value unless the prevalence is >5%.

7 Preterm deliveries

Dex is best

In the event of a possible preterm delivery parenteral maternal corticosteroid administration offers one of the most potent forms of intrauterine therapy of the neonate. In the absence of any specific data on tocolysis, the aim should be to suppress contractions long enough for the administered steroids to have their effect – that is, about 48 hours. Repeated doses and prophylactic corticosteroid administration have not been validated and there is evidence emerging that it may increase the risk of adult-onset hypertension. It is one of the most efficacious interventions in obstetrics and it should not be abused.[1]

[1]Spencer C, Neales K. Antenatal corticosteroids to prevent neonatal respiratory distress syndrome. *BMJ* 2000: **320**; 325–6.

Never do a digital when liquor is draining

This rule emphasises the importance of not performing a digital vaginal examination to assess the cervix when a woman presents with preterm rupture of the membranes. The biggest risk for the mother and baby is ascending infection and digital vaginal examinations may facilitate the ascension of vaginal microbes to cause a chorioamnionitis and enhance the onset of preterm labour. The correct and essential assessment in this situation is a speculum examination to attempt to confirm the diagnosis. A high vaginal swab should be taken to culture for *β-haemolytic streptococci* and the result must be available within 48 hours.

Exception

When an woman presents with preterm rupture of the membranes and is in active labour this rule is not valid and an assessment of the cervical dilatation and presenting part must be performed.

Meconium stained liquor and preterm labour, consider *Listeria monocytogenes*

The combination of meconium stained liquor and preterm labour is unusual and one of the possible causes is a maternal infection with *Listeria monocytogenes*, which causes fetal diarrhoea if passed on vertically by transplacental blood spread. The mother gives a history of a 'flu-like illness with or without diarrhoea. The diagnosis is confirmed with maternal blood cultures and the treatment is with high-dose intravenous ampicillin, for both the mother and the baby, and given when there is a high index of suspicion and before the culture results. Always inform the neonatal staff of your suspicions.

Deliver only when the intrauterine environment is more hostile than the neonatal unit cot

This rule states that the obstetrician should intervene in a pregnancy only when the assessments reveal that the safer option is to be delivered into a neonatal cot rather than to remain in the intrauterine environment. Generally a conservative approach should be adopted to prolong the gestation of the pregnancy as far as possible and elective delivery may be dangerous. This rule holds for most pregnancy complications like preterm rupture of the membranes, maternal hypertension, intrauterine growth restriction, antepartum haemorrhage, although the actual decision to deliver is a balanced one and should be made by the most experienced clinician after a thorough and complete assessment of the facts as we now know that the outcome for the preterm neonate is poorer when infection is present.

Avoid acidaemia at all cost

The main concept for the obstetrician with a preterm delivery is to deliver the fetus in the best possible condition for the neonatology team to deal with the problems of prematurity. Should the fetus become hypoxic and acidaemic the complications for the neonate increase dramatically. Generally preterm labours are not a problem because the labours are usually short and the delivery quick because of the small fetal head size, but the fetus must be monitored throughout. Should the labour be delayed then the obstetrician must undertake a full reassessment of the situation and consider: malpresentation (face, brow, breech or shoulder) and malposition (occipito-posterior associated with a lot of deflexion) and rarely a woman with a very small pelvis may develop an obstructed labour.

Exception

If the gestation is such that the baby is considered not viable, then monitoring should not be performed. The actual gestation will depend on the neonatal resource available at the location of the delivery. Assuming a normal baby, survival and its quality are a function of gestation and birthweight.

8
Hypertension

Never refer to the diastolic blood pressure only: "On 90"

Clinicians who refer only to the diastolic blood pressure readings ("On 90!") confirm that they understand little about the relationship between pregnancy and maternal blood pressure. It is a very bad practice that has crept into the vocabulary: it means little and should be abandoned.

As an assessment, blood pressure is one of the few objective measures in maternity care and it has two components, both of which are important. In addition, blood pressure measurements for the most part need to be interpreted in relation to a woman's non-pregnant or first trimester blood pressure. While it is true that many recognised definitions of pre-eclampsia suggest that repeated measurements of 140/90 mmHg confirm the diagnosis; equally important is the increase (delta) above the early pregnancy observations: systolic blood pressure >30 mmHg, diastolic blood pressure >15 mmHg (some say >20 mmHg). Not only will this aid the clinician in the diagnosis of pre-eclampsia in women with low non-pregnant blood pressure but may prevent unnecessary interventions late in pregnancy when physiological rises in blood pressure are commonly observed.

Exception

Obviously severe hypertension (>160/110 mmHg) requires urgent treatment with antihypertensives to protect the mother and baby.

Severe hypertension: Stabilise first, then deliver

Fulminating pre-eclampsia associated with hypertensive crisis is a medical emergency and it is very important to follow this rule. Mostly delivery will be by Caesarean section under regional anaesthesia and the patient's blood pressure must be controlled before any anaesthetic intervention. One can expect at least 48 hours' careful monitoring after delivery, including urine output, liver function tests, full blood count, and clotting studies.

Eclampsia is common postnatally and some centres recommend the use of magnesium sulphate prophylactically although the evidence for its effectiveness is still under investigation. The commonest agents used to control hypertension are intravenous hydralazine and labetolol. All are effective and use is dependent on clinical choice and experience, although intravenous labetolol appears to have less unwarranted effects.[1]

[1]Bhorat IE, Naidoo DP, Rout CC, Moodley J. Malignant ventricular arrhythmias in eclampsia: a comparison of labetolol with dihydralazine. *Am J Obstet Gynecol* 1993; **168**: 1292–6.

Systolic = maternal outcome; diastolic = fetal outcome

This rule represents another reason why clinicians should not refer to the diastolic blood pressure only. In fact it is the systolic blood pressure which reflects the maternal danger of cerebral haemorrhage and its disastrous consequences.

The mean first trimester (often mistakenly called "booking") blood pressure for a normal obstetric population is 108/66 mmHg (standard deviation = 11/8 mmHg) and a blood pressure of 140/90 mmHg is three standard deviations from the mean. The perinatal mortality is significantly increased when the diastolic reading is above 90 mmHg early in pregnancy.

The diastolic blood pressure normally drops by a mean of 15 mmHg in the second trimester. If a fall is not observed the patient is at increased risk of developing pre-eclampsia with its associated increase in perinatal morbidity and mortality.

In the third trimester blood pressure returns to early pregnancy levels by term. Clinicians need to make careful assessments of blood pressure at term to differentiate between those women who have a physiological rise in blood pressure and do not need intervention and those who have a pathological rise in blood pressure and do need interventions to deliver the baby safely.

In severe pre-eclampsia and eclampsia, do no harm and don't drown the patient

Pre-eclampsia is a disease of vasoconstriction, hypoperfusion of target organs, haemoconcentration, and increased vascular permeability which may result in total body fluid excess with intravascular fluid depletion. This makes fluid balance in these patients very difficult. Add a peripheral vasodilator like hydralazine and the fluid requirements may well be impossible to determine, but it is very important not to cause fluid overload and to wait for the natural diuresis that occurs soon after delivery.

Iatrogenic pulmonary odema and heart failure are complications that must be avoided. Central venous pressure monitoring may be helpful in anuric and/or very oedematous patients and consultation with the obstetric anaesthetist is essential.

Nothing is more important than regular careful examination of the patient's cardiovascular and respiratory systems. Heart failure can be difficult to diagnose in young women and often the only sign is a third heart sound gallop rhythm. A chest x ray and oxygen saturation monitoring may be helpful. A very safe option for fluid input is: previous hour's output plus 10–20 ml (not more than 80–100 ml per hour in the early diuretic phase).

Avoid blood transfusions for patients with severe pre-eclampsia

This is an important rule to remember as giving blood to a patient with severe pre-eclampsia may increase the intravascular oncotic pressure and may cause pulmonary odema. If at all possible leave the blood replacement until after the post-delivery diuresis has occurred.

Exception

Obviously if a patient has had acute blood loss and is anaemic then transfusion may be necessary. In such cases it should be carried out with extreme caution under control with central venous pressure monitoring.

9 Postnatal problems

Pain after birth, put your finger in first

This rule tells the obstetrician which assessment to perform in the event of a woman becoming distressed in the first 24 hours after birth with vaginal/perineal pain. More than likely the diagnosis that will be made is that of a vaginal haematoma. Sometimes the pain can be so severe that the woman will not permit the vaginal examination and any attempts will lead to profound vaginismus. The tip here is to place the woman in the left lateral position with her hips and knees well-flexed and perform the examination from the posterior aspect of the vagina.

Once the diagnosis has been confirmed it is essential to provide the patient with adequate analgesia, usually opiates and not non-steroidal anti-inflammatories (which may cause platelet dysfunction), and organise surgical drainage. Always catheterise the urinary bladder and check the haemoglobin concentration and cross-match blood for the procedure. Often the offending vessel cannot be isolated and a small corrugated drain may have to be left in the tissues for 24 hours to prevent reaccumulation.

Vaginal pain: First day, haematoma; fourth day, abscess

Following on from the above rule, if vaginal/perineal pain develops later the assessment is the same but the diagnosis is related to infection, although the initial problem may have been a small haematoma which becomes infected. The treatment intervention is surgical drainage and packing under some form of anaesthesia with healing by secondary intention, keeping the cavity clean. Sometimes delayed closure with non-absorbable sutures may be appropriate or necessary.

Cervix closed, needs antibiotics most; cervix opened, needs an operation

In the case of secondary postpartum haemorrhage the most important assessments that need to be performed are a vaginal examination and microbiological swab for culture and sensitivity testing and *not* an ultrasound scan. Cervix closed and tender uterus equals puerperal endometritis; cervix open with sub-involution of the uterus equals retained products of conception and infection. Antibiotics and bed-rest for the former and evacuation of the uterus and antibiotics for the latter.

Ultrasound imaging probably adds little and has a high false-positive rate (low specificity) which potentially leads to over-intervention. In addition, we do not know how many women with no symptoms have sonographs that are suggestive of retained products of conception. However, pelvic ultrasound scans are more helpful in management of recurrent secondary postpartum haemorrhage, in which case one should consider infection (review original swab results), placental polyps, and trophoblastic disease as possible diagnoses.

In unusual presentations after birth, consider infection first

This rule only has rare application but occasionally women may present to physicians with unusual neurological, renal or blood clotting disorder with no obvious cause in the first 4–6 weeks after birth and the obstetrician may be consulted after other medical conditions have been excluded. The usual assessments of the genital tract will identify no obvious problem like retained products of conception or endometritis and involution of the uterus is complete but the obstetrician should remember this rule.

The offending micro-organism is often an anaerobe and *Bacteroides* species may be isolated from blood cultures. Presumably the organism ascends and infects the uterine venous supply which results in a bacteraemia. Intravenous metronidazole may well have a dramatic curative effect.

Use this space to write down your own labour ward rules.

10
Conclusions

Keep your head when all about you are losing theirs

In complex and acute situations on the labour ward it is imperative that the person in charge keeps control of the situation and themselves. Panic in the voice or hands of the attendants will lose the confidence of the woman and her partner for their carers. Anxiety must be kept under control and the nervous energy transformed into action to determine the correct intervention and timing of that intervention.

Maintain control of the situation at all times.

Never compromise your professionalism

Doctors and midwives must maintain their professional standing with patients and staff alike. Honesty and integrity are qualities that must be applauded and will earn the trust and respect of those about them.

Be prepared, and do no harm

This rule applies to every obstetric intervention and especially with the advent and application of novel or new therapies.

Acknowledgements

My thanks go to Professor Phillip Baker for reading through the manuscript and offering helpful suggestions, and to Mr Lyndon Cochrane for his expert medical illustrations and patience with the author.

Use this space to write down your own labour ward rules.

Index

Page numbers in **bold** type refer to figures; those in *italic* refer to tables.

Index

Index